Breaking the Stigma
Understanding and Prioritizing Mental Health

Robert V. Hwang

Table of Contents

Chapter 1

Introduction

Mental health refers to a person's overall psychological well-being, which includes their emotional, cognitive, and social functioning. It encompasses the ability to handle stress, make meaningful connections with others, and cope with life's challenges. Good mental health is essential for individuals to achieve their full potential, maintain healthy relationships, and lead fulfilling lives. Mental health can be affected by a variety of factors, including genetics, environment, and life experiences, and can be influenced by various psychological and medical treatments. It is important to seek help if you are experiencing mental health problems, as early intervention can improve outcomes and quality of life

Definition of mental health

Mental health can be defined as a state of psychological and emotional well-being, in which an individual is able to function effectively and adapt to the demands and stresses of daily life. It involves the ability to experience a range of emotions in a healthy and balanced manner, maintain positive relationships with others, and make rational decisions. Mental health is influenced by a range of factors, including genetics, environment, social support, and access to resources and services

Mental health is a complex and dynamic aspect of human well-being that affects every area of an individual's life, including their personal relationships, work productivity, and overall quality of life. It is not just the absence of mental illness, but also the presence of positive emotions, behaviors, and attitudes that contribute to a person's overall sense of well-being.

Mental health is influenced by a range of factors, including biological, psychological, and social factors. Some of the biological factors that can affect mental health include genetics, brain chemistry, and hormonal imbalances. Psychological factors such as personality traits, coping skills, and thought patterns can also impact mental health. Social factors such as family dynamics, social support, and access to resources and services can also have a significant impact on an individual's mental health.

Mental health problems can occur at any age and can range from mild to severe. Common mental health conditions include anxiety disorders, mood disorders (such as depression and bipolar disorder), psychotic disorders (such as schizophrenia), and substance abuse disorders. These conditions can significantly affect an individual's ability to function in their daily lives and require prompt diagnosis and treatment.

It is important to prioritize mental health and engage in activities that promote well-being, such as exercise, healthy eating, and stress management techniques. Seeking professional help when needed can also be beneficial, such as counseling, therapy, or medication management. Overall, mental health is an essential aspect of

human well-being and should be given the same
level of attention and care as physical health.

Overview of the stigma surrounding mental illness

Stigma surrounding mental illness refers to
negative attitudes, beliefs, and behaviors that are
associated with mental health conditions. This
stigma can have a significant impact on
individuals who experience mental illness, their
families, and society as a whole. Stigma can lead
to discrimination, social exclusion, and limited
access to resources and services.

There are many different factors that contribute
to the stigma surrounding mental illness. One of
the main factors is a lack of understanding and
education about mental health conditions.
Misconceptions and stereotypes about mental
illness can lead to fear and misunderstanding,
and can prevent individuals from seeking help
and support.

Another factor that contributes to stigma is the way mental illness is portrayed in the media. Often, mental illness is sensationalized or portrayed in a negative light, which can perpetuate negative attitudes and beliefs.

Stigma surrounding mental illness can have significant consequences. Individuals who experience mental illness may feel ashamed or embarrassed, which can lead to social isolation and prevent them from seeking help. Stigma can also lead to discrimination in employment, housing, and other areas of life.

To address stigma surrounding mental illness, it is important to promote education and understanding about mental health conditions. This can include increasing awareness through campaigns and public events, providing accurate information about mental health, and challenging stereotypes and misconceptions.

Additionally, promoting access to resources and support can help reduce the negative impact of

stigma on individuals who experience mental
illness. This can include providing mental health
services, support groups, and other resources
that can help individuals manage their symptoms
and improve their quality of life.

Overall, addressing stigma surrounding mental
illness is an important step in promoting mental
health and well-being for all individuals

The importance of breaking the stigma
Breaking the stigma surrounding mental illness
is crucial for several reasons.

Firstly, stigma can prevent individuals who
experience mental illness from seeking help and
support. Many people who experience mental
health conditions do not seek treatment due to
fear of judgment or discrimination. This can lead
to delayed diagnosis and treatment, which can
worsen symptoms and lead to negative
outcomes.

Secondly, stigma can perpetuate negative attitudes and beliefs about mental illness, leading to discrimination and social exclusion. This can have significant consequences for individuals who experience mental illness, including difficulty finding employment, housing, and social support.

Thirdly, stigma can lead to a lack of funding and resources for mental health services and research. This can result in inadequate access to care and limited progress in developing effective treatments and interventions for mental health conditions.

By breaking the stigma surrounding mental illness, we can promote understanding and acceptance of mental health conditions. This can help individuals feel more comfortable seeking help and support, leading to earlier diagnosis and treatment. Additionally, reducing stigma can lead to increased funding and resources for mental health services and research, which can

improve outcomes for individuals who
experience mental illness.

Breaking the stigma can also lead to more
supportive and inclusive communities, where
individuals who experience mental illness are
valued and respected. This can help promote
social integration and reduce the negative impact
of discrimination and exclusion on mental
health.

Overall, breaking the stigma surrounding mental
illness is essential for promoting mental health
and well-being for all individuals. By promoting
understanding, acceptance, and support, we can
help reduce the negative impact of mental illness
on individuals, families, and society as a whole.

Chapter 2

Understanding Mental Illness

Mental illness refers to a wide range of conditions that affect a person's mood, thinking, and behavior. These conditions can significantly impact an individual's ability to function in their daily life and can range from mild to severe.

Mental illness can be caused by a variety of factors, including genetics, brain chemistry, life experiences, and environmental factors. Some common mental health conditions include anxiety disorders, mood disorders (such as depression and bipolar disorder), psychotic disorders (such as schizophrenia), and substance abuse disorders.

Symptoms of mental illness can vary depending on the condition and the individual. Common symptoms include changes in mood or behavior, difficulty concentrating, changes in appetite or sleep patterns, and feelings of hopelessness or worthlessness.

Diagnosis and treatment of mental illness typically involve a combination of therapies, including medication, psychotherapy, and lifestyle changes such as exercise and healthy eating. In some cases, hospitalization may be necessary to ensure the individual's safety and provide intensive treatment.

It is important to seek help if you or someone you know is experiencing symptoms of mental illness. Prompt diagnosis and treatment can help improve outcomes and prevent more severe symptoms from developing.

Overall, mental illness is a common and treatable condition that affects millions of individuals worldwide. By promoting understanding, acceptance, and support for individuals who experience mental illness, we can help reduce the negative impact of these conditions on individuals, families, and society as a whole.

Common mental illnesses and their symptoms
There are many different types of mental illness, each with their own set of symptoms. Here are some of the most common mental illnesses and their symptoms:

Anxiety disorders - Anxiety disorders are characterized by excessive worry, fear, and nervousness that can interfere with daily activities. Symptoms may include:
Panic attacks
- Phobias
- Obsessive-compulsive behavior
- Social anxiety
- Generalized anxiety disorder
- Mood disorders - Mood disorders are characterized by persistent feelings of sadness or extreme highs and lows. Symptoms may include:
- Depression
- Bipolar disorder
- Seasonal affective disorder

- Postpartum depression
- Personality disorders - Personality disorders are characterized by unhealthy patterns of thinking and behaving that can cause problems in relationships and daily life. Symptoms may include:
- Borderline personality disorder
- Narcissistic personality disorder
- Antisocial personality disorder
- Schizophrenia - Schizophrenia is a serious mental illness that affects a person's ability to think, feel, and behave clearly. Symptoms may include:
- Delusions
- Hallucinations
- Disorganized thinking
- Abnormal motor behavior
- Negative symptoms, such as lack of motivation or emotion
- Eating disorders - Eating disorders are characterized by extreme behaviors and attitudes towards food and weight. Symptoms may include:
- Anorexia nervosa

- Bulimia nervosa
- Binge eating disorder
- Substance abuse disorders - Substance abuse disorders are characterized by a dependence on drugs or alcohol. Symptoms may include:
- Withdrawal symptoms
- Cravings
- Physical dependence
- Tolerance

These are just a few of the many types of mental illness and their symptoms. If you or someone you know is experiencing any of these symptoms, it is important to seek help from a mental health professional

Myths and misconceptions surrounding mental illness

There are many myths and misconceptions surrounding mental illness. Here are some of the most common:

- Mental illness is a personal weakness or character flaw. In reality, mental illness is a medical condition that is caused by a variety of factors, including genetics, brain chemistry, and life experiences.

- People with mental illness are violent and dangerous. This is a harmful stereotype that is not supported by research. In fact, people with mental illness are more likely to be victims of violence than perpetrators.
- Mental illness is a rare condition. Mental illness is actually very common, with one in four adults experiencing a mental health condition in any given year.
- Mental illness is a lifelong condition that cannot be treated. While some mental health conditions may be chronic, many can be effectively treated with medication, therapy, and lifestyle changes.
- Mental illness only affects certain types of people. Mental illness can affect anyone, regardless of age, gender, race, or socioeconomic status.
- People with mental illness should just "snap out of it" or "get over it." Mental

illness is a medical condition that requires professional treatment and support.

These myths and misconceptions can prevent people from seeking help and support for mental illness, leading to delayed diagnosis and treatment. By promoting understanding and acceptance of mental illness, we can help reduce the negative impact of these misconceptions and promote better mental health for all

The biological and environmental factors contributing to mental illness

Mental illness is a complex condition that can be caused by a variety of factors, both biological and environmental. Here are some of the key factors that contribute to mental illness:

- Genetics: Genetics can play a role in the development of mental illness. Some mental health conditions, such as bipolar disorder and schizophrenia, are known to have a genetic component.

- Brain chemistry: Neurotransmitters, the chemicals that regulate communication between brain cells, can be imbalanced in individuals with mental illness. For example, low levels of serotonin are associated with depression.
- Trauma: Traumatic events, such as abuse or neglect, can increase the risk of developing mental illness.
- Environmental stressors: Chronic stress from factors such as poverty, discrimination, or unemployment can contribute to the development of mental illness.
- Substance abuse: Substance abuse can alter brain chemistry and increase the risk of developing mental health conditions such as depression and anxiety.
- Medical conditions: Certain medical conditions, such as chronic pain or cancer, can increase the risk of developing mental health conditions.

It's important to note that mental illness is often caused by a combination of factors, and not just one single cause. Additionally, not everyone who experiences these risk factors will develop mental illness, and some individuals may develop mental illness without any known risk factors.

Understanding the complex interplay between biological and environmental factors can help individuals and their healthcare providers identify potential risk factors and develop effective treatment plans. By addressing both the biological and environmental factors contributing to mental illness, individuals can achieve better mental health outcomes

Chapter 3

The Impact of Stigma

Stigma surrounding mental illness can have a significant impact on individuals, families, and communities. The impact of stigma surrounding mental illness can be far-reaching and can affect not only individuals with mental illness but also their families and communities. Here are some of the ways stigma can impact those with mental illness:

- Lack of understanding and awareness: Stigma can lead to a lack of understanding and awareness about mental illness. This can prevent individuals from recognizing the signs and symptoms of mental illness in themselves or others, leading to delayed diagnosis and treatment.
- Internalized shame and self-stigma: Stigma can cause individuals with mental illness to internalize shame and self-stigma. They may believe they are weak, flawed, or defective, leading to feelings of low self-worth and self-esteem.
- Reduced access to resources: Stigma can limit access to mental health resources and support systems. Individuals may be hesitant to seek help from healthcare providers or support groups due to fear of judgment or discrimination.

- Inadequate healthcare: Stigma can lead to inadequate healthcare for individuals with mental illness. Healthcare providers may not take their symptoms seriously, leading to misdiagnosis, delayed treatment, or inappropriate treatment.
- Negative impact on families: Stigma can also have a negative impact on families of individuals with mental illness. They may experience feelings of shame,embarrassment, or guilt, which can lead to isolation and a lack of support.
- Barriers to treatment: Stigma can prevent individuals with mental illness from seeking help and treatment. They may fear being judged, discriminated against, or shamed for their condition, leading to delayed diagnosis and treatment.
- Social isolation: Stigma can cause individuals with mental illness to feel isolated and alone. They may withdraw from social activities or avoid seeking help, leading to increased feelings of loneliness and despair.

- Employment discrimination: Stigma can lead to employment discrimination against individuals with mental illness. Employers may be reluctant to hire or promote individuals with mental illness, even if they are capable of performing their job duties.
- Financial burden: Stigma can also lead to financial burden for individuals with mental illness. Treatment and therapy may be costly, and individuals may face additional expenses such as transportation costs to attend appointments.
- Negative stereotypes: Stigma can perpetuate negative stereotypes about individuals with mental illness. This can lead to discrimination, harassment, and bullying, which can further isolate individuals and exacerbate their mental health condition.

Breaking down the stigma surrounding mental illness is essential for promoting understanding, acceptance, and access to care. By reducing stigma, individuals with mental illness can seek help without fear of judgment, and communities can provide support and resources to those in need. This can lead to better mental health outcomes for everyone

The effects of stigma on mental health
Stigma surrounding mental illness can have negative effects on mental health. Here are some of the ways stigma can impact mental health:

- Substance use: Stigma can increase the risk of substance use among individuals with mental illness. They may turn to drugs or alcohol to cope with the negative emotions and stress caused by stigma and discrimination.
- Disengagement from treatment: Stigma can cause individuals with mental illness to disengage from treatment. They may feel that seeking help is pointless due to the negative attitudes and beliefs surrounding mental illness, leading to a

lack of follow-up care and medication adherence.

- Impact on physical health: Stigma can also impact physical health. Individuals with mental illness may experience physical symptoms such as headaches, muscle tension, and fatigue due to the stress caused by stigma.
- Interpersonal relationships: Stigma can impact interpersonal relationships for individuals with mental illness. They may face rejection, discrimination, or social exclusion, leading to a lack of social support and a further decline in mental health.
- Reduced employment opportunities: Stigma can limit employment opportunities for individuals with mental illness, leading to financial strain and a reduced sense of purpose and self-worth.
- Increased stress: Stigma can lead to increased stress, which can exacerbate mental health conditions. Individuals may experience discrimination, bullying, or

harassment due to their mental illness, leading to increased feelings of anxiety and depression.

- Self-stigma: Stigma can cause individuals with mental illness to internalize negative beliefs and stereotypes about themselves, leading to self-stigma. This can lead to feelings of shame, guilt, and low self-esteem, which can further exacerbate mental health conditions.
- Delayed treatment: Stigma can prevent individuals from seeking help for mental health conditions, leading to delayed treatment. This can lead to worsening symptoms and a longer recovery time.
- Reduced quality of care: Stigma can also lead to reduced quality of care for individuals with mental illness. Healthcare providers may not take their symptoms seriously, leading to misdiagnosis, delayed treatment, or inappropriate treatment.
- Social isolation: Stigma can cause individuals with mental illness to feel isolated and alone. They may withdraw

from social activities or avoid seeking
help, leading to increased feelings of
loneliness and despair.
- Suicide risk: Stigma can increase the risk
of suicide among individuals with mental
illness. Individuals may feel hopeless,
helpless, and alone, leading to an
increased risk of suicidal ideation and
attempts.

Breaking down stigma surrounding mental illness is essential for promoting mental health and well-being. By reducing stigma, individuals can seek help without fear of judgment or discrimination, leading to earlier diagnosis and treatment. This can help improve mental health outcomes and prevent negative effects of stigma on mental health

How stigma can prevent people from seeking help

Stigma surrounding mental illness can prevent people from seeking help in several ways:

- Fear of judgment: Individuals may fear being judged or discriminated against if they seek help for mental health issues. They may worry about being seen as weak or incompetent, leading them to avoid seeking help altogether.
- Self-stigma: Stigma can also lead to self-stigma, where individuals internalize negative beliefs and stereotypes about mental illness. They may feel ashamed or guilty about their condition and avoid seeking help due to a belief that they are not deserving of care.
- Lack of awareness: Stigma can also contribute to a lack of awareness about mental health issues. Individuals may not realize that their symptoms are indicative of a mental health condition or may believe that seeking help is unnecessary.
- Social pressure: Stigma can also create social pressure to conform to certain beliefs or attitudes about mental illness. Individuals may feel that seeking help for mental health issues is taboo or seen as a

weakness, leading them to avoid seeking help altogether.

- Limited access to care: Stigma can also contribute to limited access to care for mental health issues. Healthcare providers may be reluctant to diagnose or treat mental illness due to stigma, or individuals may face financial or logistical barriers to accessing care.

Breaking down stigma surrounding mental illness is essential for promoting mental health and well-being. By reducing stigma, individuals can feel more comfortable seeking help and receive appropriate treatment and support. This can help to prevent the negative effects of mental illness and improve overall well-being.

The social and economic costs of mental illness stigma

Stigma surrounding mental illness can have significant social and economic costs. Here are some examples:

- Reduced productivity: Mental illness stigma can reduce productivity in the workplace, leading to decreased efficiency, absenteeism, and presenteeism. This can result in significant economic costs for employers and society as a whole.
- Increased healthcare costs: Stigma can increase healthcare costs by reducing the likelihood that individuals with mental illness will seek help for their condition. This can lead to delayed diagnosis and treatment, which can result in more severe symptoms and complications, ultimately leading to higher healthcare costs.
- Social isolation: Stigma can lead to social isolation and exclusion for individuals with mental illness. This can result in a lack of social support, which can

exacerbate symptoms and contribute to a decline in mental health.

- Discrimination: Stigma can contribute to discrimination against individuals with mental illness, leading to negative attitudes and behaviors from others, including employers, healthcare providers, and the general public.
- Limited access to care: Stigma can also contribute to limited access to care for mental health issues, leading to a lack of appropriate treatment and support. This can result in more severe symptoms and complications, leading to increased healthcare costs and decreased productivity.

Overall, the social and economic costs of mental illness stigma can be significant, highlighting the importance of reducing stigma and promoting mental health and well-being for all individuals.

Chapter 4

Challenging Stigma

Challenging stigma surrounding mental illness is essential for promoting mental health and well-being. Here are some ways that individuals and communities can challenge stigma:

- Education and awareness: Education and awareness about mental illness can help to challenge stigma. By increasing knowledge and understanding of mental illness, individuals can break down stereotypes and reduce discrimination.
- Language use: Language use can also impact stigma surrounding mental illness. Avoiding derogatory terms and using person-first language (e.g., "person with bipolar disorder" instead of "bipolar person") can help to reduce stigma and promote a more respectful and empathetic view of mental illness.
- Encouraging open discussion: Encouraging open discussion about

mental illness can help to break down stigma. By creating a safe space for individuals to share their experiences and seek support, individuals can feel more comfortable seeking help and discussing their mental health.

- Challenging stereotypes: Challenging stereotypes and negative beliefs about mental illness can also help to break down stigma. By highlighting the diversity of experiences and challenges faced by individuals with mental illness, individuals can break down assumptions and misconceptions.
- Advocacy and policy change: Advocacy and policy change can also contribute to reducing stigma. By advocating for changes in healthcare policies and practices, individuals can ensure that mental health is prioritized and that individuals with mental illness receive appropriate care and support.

Challenging stigma surrounding mental illness is crucial for promoting mental health and well-being for all individuals. By working together to break down stereotypes and promote understanding, individuals can help to create a more accepting and supportive society for individuals with mental illness

Strategies for challenging mental illness stigma at the individual level
Challenging mental illness stigma at the individual level can be a powerful way to promote understanding and acceptance. Here are some strategies for challenging mental illness stigma at the individual level:

- Educate yourself: Educating yourself about mental illness can help to challenge stigma. Read books, articles, and other resources that provide accurate information about mental illness, including its causes, symptoms, and treatment options.

- Challenge your own biases: Everyone has biases, and it's important to be aware of them. Challenge your own biases about mental illness and work to develop a more open and empathetic perspective.
- Speak up: Speak up when you hear someone making derogatory comments about mental illness. Explain why such comments are hurtful and challenge stereotypes and misconceptions.
- Use person-first language: Using person-first language (e.g., "person with depression" instead of "depressed person") can help to promote a more respectful and empathetic view of mental illness.
- Share your story: Sharing your own experiences with mental illness can help to break down stigma and encourage others to seek help. By talking openly about your own struggles and successes, you can help to create a more accepting and supportive environment for individuals with mental illness.

- Support individuals with mental illness: Show support for individuals with mental illness by listening to them, providing encouragement, and helping them to access appropriate care and support.

By challenging mental illness stigma at the individual level, we can create a more accepting and supportive society for individuals with mental illness. Each of us has a role to play in reducing stigma and promoting understanding, and by working together, we can make a difference

The role of family and community in reducing stigma

Family and community play a crucial role in reducing stigma surrounding mental illness. Here are some ways that family and community can contribute to reducing stigma:

- Education and awareness: Family and community can help to reduce stigma by increasing knowledge and awareness of mental illness. By educating themselves and others about mental illness, family and community members can break down stereotypes and reduce discrimination.

- Support: Family and community support is essential for individuals with mental illness. Providing emotional and practical support can help to reduce feelings of isolation and encourage individuals to seek help when needed.
- Advocacy: Family and community members can also advocate for changes in policies and practices that impact individuals with mental illness. By advocating for improved access to mental health care and reduced discrimination, family and community members can help to promote a more supportive and accepting environment for individuals with mental illness.
- Open communication: Encouraging open communication about mental illness can help to reduce stigma. Family and community members can create safe spaces for individuals with mental illness

to discuss their experiences and seek support without fear of judgment or discrimination.

- Challenging stereotypes: Family and community members can challenge stereotypes and negative beliefs about mental illness. By highlighting the diversity of experiences and challenges faced by individuals with mental illness, family and community members can break down assumptions and misconceptions.

Reducing stigma surrounding mental illness requires a collective effort from all members of society, including family and community. By working together to promote understanding and acceptance of mental illness, we can create a more supportive and inclusive environment for individuals with mental illness

Advocacy and policy interventions to reduce stigma

Advocacy and policy interventions are essential to reducing stigma surrounding mental illness. Here are some examples of advocacy and policy interventions that can be effective in reducing stigma:

- Anti-stigma campaigns: Anti-stigma campaigns are an effective way to increase awareness and understanding of mental illness. These campaigns can use a variety of media and outreach methods, such as social media, television ads, and community events.
- Training programs: Training programs for healthcare providers, educators, and other professionals can help to reduce stigma by increasing knowledge and awareness of mental illness. These programs can include information on best practices for treating individuals with mental illness and strategies for reducing stigma in the workplace.
- Legislation and policy changes: Legislation and policy changes can help to

reduce stigma by promoting access to mental health services and reducing discrimination. Examples of policy changes include laws that prohibit discrimination against individuals with mental illness in the workplace or in housing.

- Funding for mental health services: Increased funding for mental health services can help to reduce stigma by improving access to care and reducing barriers to treatment. This can include funding for community mental health centers, crisis hotlines, and other resources.
- Advocacy for mental health parity: Advocacy for mental health parity can help to reduce stigma by ensuring that mental health services are covered by insurance at the same level as physical health services. This can include advocating for laws that require insurance companies to provide equal coverage for mental and physical health services.

Reducing stigma surrounding mental illness requires a coordinated effort that involves advocacy, policy interventions, and community engagement. By working together to promote understanding and acceptance of mental illness, we can create a more supportive and inclusive environment for individuals with mental illness.

Chapter 5

Prioritizing Mental Health

Prioritizing mental health is essential for promoting overall well-being and improving quality of life for individuals and communities. Prioritizing mental health requires a multifaceted approach that involves education, access to services, prevention, integration of care, and support for caregivers. By prioritizing mental health, we can create a more supportive and inclusive environment for individuals with mental illness and promote overall well-being in our communities.

The importance of self-care for mental health
Self-care is critical for promoting mental health and well-being. It involves taking deliberate actions to care for one's physical, emotional, and mental health. Here are some ways that self-care can benefit mental health:

- Reducing stress: Stress can contribute to the development of mental health problems such as anxiety and depression. Engaging in self-care activities such as exercise, meditation, or spending time in nature can help to reduce stress levels.

- Improving mood: Self-care activities can also help to improve mood and increase feelings of happiness and well-being. This can include engaging in hobbies or activities that bring joy, spending time with loved ones, or engaging in self-compassion practices.
- Building resilience: Self-care can also help to build resilience and increase the ability to cope with difficult situations. This can include engaging in activities that promote self-reflection and personal growth, such as journaling or therapy.
- Enhancing self-esteem: Engaging in self-care activities can help to enhance self-esteem and self-worth. This can include engaging in activities that promote self-acceptance, self-love, and self-compassion.

- Improving overall health: Self-care can also improve overall health, which can have a positive impact on mental health. This can include engaging in regular exercise, eating a healthy diet, and getting enough sleep.

Creating supportive environments for mental health

Creating supportive environments for mental health is critical for promoting overall well-being and reducing the impact of mental illness on individuals and communities. Here are some ways that supportive environments can be created:

- Reduce stigma and discrimination: Reducing stigma and discrimination surrounding mental illness is critical for creating a supportive environment. This can include increasing education and awareness about mental health issues, providing resources for individuals with mental illness, and promoting acceptance and understanding.

- Increase access to mental health services: Ensuring access to mental health services is essential for promoting mental health. This can include increasing funding for mental health services, providing mental health resources in community settings, and improving insurance coverage for mental health services.

- Create safe and supportive spaces: Creating safe and supportive spaces where individuals feel comfortable discussing mental health issues can help to reduce stigma and promote understanding. This can include creating support groups, providing mental health resources in workplaces and schools, and promoting mental health awareness campaigns.

- Encourage self-care: Encouraging self-care and wellness practices can promote mental health and well-being. This can include promoting physical activity, healthy eating, and stress reduction techniques such as meditation or yoga.

- Foster social connections: Fostering social connections can help to promote mental health and reduce social isolation. This can include creating opportunities for social interaction, promoting community involvement, and providing resources for individuals who may be at risk of social isolation.

Creating supportive environments for mental health requires a multifaceted approach that involves reducing stigma, increasing access to services, creating safe and supportive spaces, encouraging self-care, and fostering social connections. By prioritizing mental health and creating supportive environments, we can promote overall well-being and reduce the impact of mental illness on individuals and communities.

Access to mental health services and resources

Access to mental health services and resources is critical for promoting mental health and well-being. Here are some ways to increase access:

- Increase funding for mental health services: One way to increase access to mental health services is to increase funding for mental health programs and services. This can include funding for community mental health centers, school-based mental health programs, and mental health research.
- Improve insurance coverage: Another way to increase access to mental health services is to improve insurance coverage for mental health care. This can include requiring insurance companies to cover mental health care at the same level as physical health care, and expanding Medicaid coverage to cover more mental health services.
- Promote telehealth and online resources: Telehealth and online resources can

increase access to mental health services, especially for individuals who live in rural or remote areas. This can include teletherapy sessions, online mental health resources, and mobile apps designed to support mental health.

- Increase availability of mental health services in schools and workplaces: Increasing the availability of mental health services in schools and workplaces can help to reduce barriers to accessing care. This can include providing mental health resources in employee wellness programs and offering mental health services in schools.

- Train primary care providers: Primary care providers can play a critical role in identifying and treating mental health issues. Providing training for primary care providers on how to recognize and treat mental health issues can increase access to care for individuals who may not seek care from a mental health specialist.

Increasing access to mental health services and resources is critical for promoting mental health and well-being. By increasing funding for mental health services, improving insurance coverage, promoting telehealth and online resources, increasing availability of mental health services in schools and workplaces, and training primary care providers, we can improve access to care and reduce barriers to treatment.

Chapter 6

Social Determinants of Mental Health

Social determinants are the conditions in which people are born, grow, live, work, and age that affect their health and well-being. Social determinants of mental health are the social and economic factors that influence mental health outcomes. Here are some examples of social determinants of mental health:

- Poverty: Poverty is a significant social determinant of mental health. Individuals who live in poverty are at increased risk for mental health problems due to factors such as chronic stress, inadequate nutrition, and limited access to healthcare.

- Education: Education is another social determinant of mental health. Higher levels of education are associated with better mental health outcomes, as education can provide individuals with better job opportunities, higher income, and a sense of purpose and meaning.
- Social support: Social support is critical for mental health, and lack of social support is a social determinant of mental health. Individuals who have strong social connections and support networks are less likely to experience mental health problems.
- Discrimination: Discrimination based on race, ethnicity, gender, sexual orientation, or other factors is a significant social determinant of mental health. Discrimination can lead to chronic stress and trauma, which can contribute to mental health problems.

- Housing: Housing is a social determinant of mental health, as inadequate housing can contribute to stress, insecurity, and social isolation. Individuals who are homeless or live in unstable housing situations are at increased risk for mental health problems.
- Access to healthcare: Access to healthcare is a social determinant of mental health. Individuals who have limited access to healthcare, including mental health services, are at increased risk for mental health problems.

Understanding the social determinants of mental health is critical for promoting mental health and well-being. Addressing social determinants of mental health requires a comprehensive approach that involves improving access to healthcare, addressing poverty and inequality, promoting social support and connectedness, and addressing discrimination and stigma. By addressing social determinants of mental health, we can promote overall well-being and reduce the impact of mental illness on individuals and communities.

The impact of social determinants on mental health

Social determinants of mental health can significantly impact individuals' mental health outcomes. Here are some of the ways social determinants can affect mental health:

- Poverty: Living in poverty can increase the risk of developing mental health problems, including depression and anxiety. Poverty can cause chronic stress, which can lead to poor mental health outcomes.
- Education: Education is a social determinant of mental health, as individuals with higher levels of education are less likely to experience mental health problems. Education can provide individuals with better job opportunities, higher income, and a sense of purpose and meaning.

- Social support: Social support is critical for mental health, and lack of social support is a social determinant of mental health. Individuals who have strong social connections and support networks are less likely to experience mental health problems.
- Discrimination: Discrimination can lead to chronic stress and trauma, which can contribute to mental health problems. Discrimination based on race, ethnicity, gender, sexual orientation, or other factors is a significant social determinant of mental health.
- Housing: Housing is a social determinant of mental health, as inadequate housing can contribute to stress, insecurity, and social isolation. Individuals who are homeless or live in unstable housing situations are at increased risk for mental health problems.
- Access to healthcare: Access to healthcare is a social determinant of mental health. Individuals who have limited access to

healthcare, including mental health services, are at increased risk for mental health problems.

Understanding the impact of social determinants on mental health is essential for promoting mental health and well-being. Addressing social determinants of mental health requires a comprehensive approach that involves improving access to healthcare, addressing poverty and inequality, promoting social support and connectedness, and addressing discrimination and stigma. By addressing social determinants of mental health, we can promote overall well-being and reduce the impact of mental illness on individuals and communities.

Addressing social determinants through policy and advocacy
Addressing social determinants of mental health through policy and advocacy is essential to improve mental health outcomes for individuals and communities. Here are some ways policy

and advocacy can address social determinants of mental health:

- Healthcare reform: Healthcare reform can address social determinants of mental health by expanding access to mental health services and integrating mental health care into primary care. Healthcare reform can also address disparities in access to healthcare based on race, ethnicity, income, and other factors.
- Poverty reduction: Addressing poverty through policies such as raising the minimum wage, expanding access to affordable housing, and providing access to social safety net programs can reduce the impact of poverty on mental health.
- Education reform: Education reform can address social determinants of mental health by improving access to education and promoting education policies that reduce disparities in access to education based on race, income, and other factors.

- Anti-discrimination policies: Policies that address discrimination based on race, ethnicity, gender, sexual orientation, and other factors can reduce the impact of discrimination on mental health.
- Community-based programs: Community-based programs that promote social support and connectedness can address social determinants of mental health by addressing social isolation and promoting social connectedness.
- Mental health awareness campaigns: Mental health awareness campaigns can address stigma and discrimination by promoting mental health literacy and reducing the stigma associated with mental illness.

By addressing social determinants of mental health through policy and advocacy, we can improve mental health outcomes and promote overall well-being for individuals and communities. Advocacy efforts should prioritize the needs of marginalized and underserved communities to ensure that policies and programs are equitable and address the root causes of mental health disparities

The role of community-based organizations in promoting mental health.
Community-based organizations (CBOs) play a vital role in promoting mental health by providing support and resources to individuals and communities. Here are some ways CBOs can promote mental health:

- Education and awareness: CBOs can provide education and awareness campaigns on mental health issues and reduce the stigma surrounding mental illness. This can help to increase mental health literacy and reduce barriers to seeking help.
- Support groups: CBOs can provide support groups for individuals with mental health challenges, such as depression, anxiety, and trauma. These groups provide a safe and supportive environment for

individuals to share their experiences and receive emotional support.

- Advocacy: CBOs can advocate for policies and programs that promote mental health and address social determinants of mental health. This includes advocating for access to mental health services, reducing stigma, and promoting social and economic policies that support mental health.
- Skill-building: CBOs can provide skill-building programs that promote resilience and coping strategies. This can include stress-management techniques, mindfulness, and other self-care practices.
- Community engagement: CBOs can engage community members in mental health promotion efforts. This can include community events and activities that promote mental health, such as walks and workshops.

By providing these resources and services, CBOs can help to promote mental health and improve the overall well-being of individuals and communities. Additionally, CBOs can play a critical role in addressing mental health disparities by prioritizing the needs of marginalized and underserved communities.

Chapter 7

Promoting Mental Wellness

Promoting mental wellness involves taking proactive steps to maintain good mental health and prevent mental health challenges. Here are some strategies for promoting mental wellness:

- Self-care: Practicing self-care can help promote mental wellness. This includes getting enough sleep, eating a healthy diet, engaging in regular exercise, and finding time for relaxation and leisure activities.
- Social connections: Having social connections and support systems can help promote mental wellness. This includes maintaining relationships with friends and family, joining clubs or groups that share your interests, and seeking out community resources and services.
- Positive thinking: Developing a positive mindset and focusing on positive aspects of your life can promote mental wellness. This can include practicing gratitude,

affirmations, and reframing negative thoughts.

- Learning new skills: Engaging in activities that challenge you and promote personal growth can promote mental wellness. This can include learning a new language, taking up a new hobby, or engaging in creative activities.
- Seeking help when needed: Seeking help when experiencing mental health challenges is an important part of promoting mental wellness. This includes seeking support from a mental health professional, talking to a trusted friend or family member, or accessing community resources and services.

Promoting mental wellness is important for overall health and well-being. By taking proactive steps to maintain good mental health, individuals can prevent mental health challenges and improve their quality of life.

Evidence-based interventions for promoting mental wellness

There are several evidence-based interventions for promoting mental wellness. Here are some examples:

- Cognitive-behavioral therapy (CBT): CBT is a type of therapy that helps individuals identify and change negative thought patterns and behaviors that contribute to mental health challenges. It is effective in treating conditions such as depression and anxiety.
- Mindfulness-based interventions: Mindfulness-based interventions, such as mindfulness meditation and mindfulness-based stress reduction, are effective in reducing stress and promoting overall well-being.

- Physical exercise: Regular exercise has been shown to have a positive impact on mental health by reducing symptoms of depression and anxiety and improving overall mood.
- Social support: Having social support is important for promoting mental wellness. Interventions that focus on building social connections and support networks, such as support groups and peer-to-peer counseling, can be effective.
- Nutrition interventions: Interventions that focus on promoting a healthy diet, such as the Mediterranean diet, have been shown to have a positive impact on mental health.
- Resilience-building interventions: Interventions that focus on promoting resilience, such as stress-management techniques and coping skills, can help individuals better manage stress and prevent mental health challenges.

These interventions have been shown to be effective in promoting mental wellness and preventing mental health challenges. By incorporating these interventions into daily life, individuals can improve their overall well-being and promote mental wellness.

The importance of early intervention and prevention

Early intervention and prevention are crucial for promoting mental health and preventing mental health challenges. Here are some reasons why early intervention and prevention are important:

1. Early intervention can prevent mental health challenges from becoming more severe. By addressing mental health challenges early on, individuals can avoid the negative consequences that may result from untreated or poorly managed mental health conditions.
2. Early intervention can improve outcomes. Research has shown that early intervention can lead to better outcomes

for individuals with mental health challenges, such as improved symptom management, increased functioning, and better quality of life.

3. Prevention can reduce the risk of developing mental health challenges. By identifying risk factors and implementing prevention strategies, individuals can reduce their risk of developing mental health challenges in the first place.

4. Prevention can improve overall well-being. Prevention strategies, such as practicing self-care and stress-management techniques, can promote overall well-being and help individuals manage stress and other challenges before they develop into mental health conditions.

5. Early intervention and prevention can reduce the economic burden of mental health challenges. By addressing mental health challenges early on and implementing prevention strategies, individuals can reduce the economic

burden of mental health challenges on themselves, their families, and society as a whole.

Overall, early intervention and prevention are important for promoting mental health and preventing mental health challenges. By taking proactive steps to address mental health challenges early on and prevent them from occurring in the first place, individuals can improve their overall well-being and quality of life

Promoting mental wellness in schools, workplaces, and other settings
Promoting mental wellness in schools, workplaces, and other settings is crucial for supporting the mental health of individuals in these environments. Here are some ways that mental wellness can be promoted in these settings:

- Schools: Schools can promote mental wellness by creating a safe and supportive learning environment for students. This can include providing access to mental health resources and support services, promoting positive coping skills and stress management techniques, and creating a culture of inclusivity and acceptance.

- Workplaces: Workplaces can promote mental wellness by creating a culture of mental health awareness and support. This can include providing access to mental health resources and support services, promoting work-life balance and stress management techniques, and fostering a culture of open communication and support.
- Other settings: Mental wellness can be promoted in other settings, such as community centers, religious institutions, and recreational facilities, by providing access to mental health resources and support services, promoting positive coping skills and stress management techniques, and fostering a culture of inclusivity and acceptance.

Some specific strategies for promoting mental wellness in these settings may include:

- Providing access to mental health resources and support services, such as counseling and therapy, support groups, and mental health hotlines.
- Offering training and education for individuals to develop skills for managing stress, anxiety, and other mental health challenges.
- Promoting work-life balance by encouraging flexible scheduling, setting realistic workloads, and promoting healthy lifestyle habits.
- Creating a culture of inclusivity and acceptance by promoting diversity, equity, and inclusion.
- Encouraging open communication and support by providing opportunities for individuals to connect with one another and share their experiences.

Overall, promoting mental wellness in schools, workplaces, and other settings is important for supporting the mental health of individuals and creating a culture of well-being and support.

Chapter 8

The Intersection of Mental Health and Social Justice

The intersection of mental health and social justice is an important area of study and practice that focuses on understanding the ways in which social inequality and oppression can negatively impact mental health and wellbeing.

Social justice refers to the idea that everyone should have equal rights, opportunities, and access to resources and that systemic barriers to equality must be dismantled. In the context of mental health, social justice advocates for ensuring that all individuals have access to quality mental health care and support, regardless of their race, gender, socioeconomic status, or other marginalized identities.

The relationship between mental health and social justice is complex and multifaceted. Marginalized individuals and communities often experience higher rates of mental health issues, such as anxiety, depression, and post-traumatic stress disorder (PTSD), due to the impact of systemic oppression and discrimination on their lives. These factors can lead to increased stress, trauma, and feelings of hopelessness and helplessness, which can in turn negatively affect mental health.

At the same time, mental health issues can also contribute to social inequality and injustice. For example, individuals with mental health issues may face stigma, discrimination, and unequal treatment in education, employment, and housing. Additionally, access to quality mental health care and support may be limited for individuals with marginalized identities, further perpetuating inequalities.

To address the intersection of mental health and social justice, it is important to take a holistic approach that considers the social determinants of mental health and the systemic barriers to mental health care and support. This includes addressing issues such as poverty, racism, sexism, and ableism, as well as ensuring that mental health services are accessible and culturally competent for all individuals. By addressing these issues, we can work towards creating a more equitable and just society that promotes the mental health and wellbeing of all individuals.

The impact of systemic oppression on mental health

Systemic oppression can have a significant impact on mental health. Oppression refers to the systemic and institutionalized mistreatment of individuals and groups based on their race, gender, sexual orientation, religion, socioeconomic status, and other marginalized identities. The experience of oppression can lead to a range of mental health issues, including anxiety, depression, post-traumatic stress disorder (PTSD), and other stress-related disorders.

One way in which systemic oppression can impact mental health is through the experience of microaggressions. Microaggressions are subtle forms of discrimination that are often unintentional but can still have harmful effects on individuals. These can include comments, gestures, or behaviors that are derogatory or demeaning towards individuals based on their marginalized identity. The experience of microaggressions can lead to feelings of isolation, self-doubt, and anxiety, which can contribute to mental health issues.

Systemic oppression can also impact mental health by limiting access to resources and opportunities. For example, individuals who experience discrimination and oppression may face barriers to education, employment, and healthcare. This lack of access to basic resources can contribute to feelings of hopelessness and helplessness, which can negatively impact mental health.

Moreover, the experience of systemic oppression can lead to trauma, which can have a lasting impact on mental health. Trauma can result from experiencing or witnessing events that threaten one's physical or emotional safety. Examples of traumatic experiences can include police brutality, hate crimes, and discrimination in the workplace or education system. The impact of trauma on mental health can include symptoms such as flashbacks, nightmares, and hyper-vigilance.

Overall, the impact of systemic oppression on mental health is significant and requires attention from mental health professionals, policy-makers, and advocates for social justice. It is essential to address systemic oppression and work towards creating a more equitable society to promote the mental health and wellbeing of all individuals

The importance of addressing social justice in mental health advocacy

Addressing social justice is essential in mental health advocacy because social inequalities and injustices have a significant impact on mental health. Individuals who belong to marginalized groups, such as people of color, LGBTQ+ individuals, and those living in poverty, are at a higher risk of developing mental health issues due to systemic oppression and discrimination. Addressing social justice issues is therefore critical to promoting mental health and wellbeing for all individuals, regardless of their background or identity.

Mental health advocacy efforts that focus solely on individual-level interventions, such as therapy and medication, may not be effective in addressing the root causes of mental health issues. Social justice advocates for a more comprehensive approach that addresses the underlying social determinants of mental health, including poverty, racism, sexism, and ableism. This involves promoting policies and programs that address these issues, such as increasing access to affordable housing, improving access to healthcare, and reducing discrimination in the workplace and education system.

Additionally, mental health advocacy efforts that ignore social justice issues may perpetuate inequalities and contribute to the marginalization of already vulnerable populations. For example, mental health services that are not culturally competent and do not take into account the experiences of marginalized individuals may further stigmatize and alienate these populations, reducing their willingness to seek help.

By addressing social justice issues in mental health advocacy, we can work towards creating a more equitable and just society that promotes the mental health and wellbeing of all individuals. This requires a multi-faceted approach that addresses the root causes of mental health issues and promotes access to resources and support for all individuals, regardless of their background or identity.

The role of mental health professionals in promoting social justice

Mental health professionals can play a critical role in promoting social justice by advocating for their clients and addressing the systemic and institutional barriers that can impact their mental health. This involves understanding the ways in which social inequalities and injustices can impact mental health, and working towards creating a more equitable and just society.

One way in which mental health professionals can promote social justice is by addressing issues of power and privilege in their work. This includes recognizing the ways in which their own social identities and experiences may impact their interactions with clients and addressing any biases or assumptions they may hold. It also involves empowering clients to assert their own needs and advocating for them in situations where they may face discrimination or unequal treatment.

Mental health professionals can also advocate for policy changes that address social justice issues related to mental health. This can include advocating for increased funding for mental health services, promoting policies that reduce discrimination and bias in healthcare settings, and supporting efforts to address the social determinants of mental health, such as poverty and access to education.

Additionally, mental health professionals can work towards creating more inclusive and culturally competent mental health services that address the unique needs of individuals from diverse backgrounds. This involves understanding the ways in which cultural beliefs and practices can impact mental health, and developing interventions that are culturally sensitive and responsive to the needs of diverse populations.

Overall, mental health professionals have a critical role to play in promoting social justice and addressing the root causes of mental health issues. By recognizing the impact of systemic oppression and working towards creating a more equitable and just society, mental health professionals can promote the mental health and wellbeing of all individuals, regardless of their background or identity

Chapter 9

Moving Forward

Moving forward, it is important to continue addressing the intersection of mental health and social justice. This includes recognizing the ways in which systemic oppression and discrimination can impact mental health, and working towards creating a more equitable and just society that promotes the mental health and wellbeing of all individuals.

One way to address these issues is through education and awareness-raising efforts. Mental health professionals, policy-makers, and advocates for social justice can work together to promote a better understanding of the ways in which social inequalities and injustices can impact mental health, and to develop strategies to address these issues.

Another important step is to increase access to mental health services for marginalized populations. This involves addressing the barriers that can prevent individuals from seeking help, such as stigma, lack of resources, and discrimination in healthcare settings. It also requires developing interventions that are culturally competent and responsive to the unique needs of diverse populations.

Furthermore, it is important to advocate for policy changes that address the root causes of mental health issues, such as poverty, discrimination, and unequal access to resources. This includes promoting policies that address the social determinants of mental health, such as access to education, employment, and healthcare.

Overall, addressing the intersection of mental health and social justice requires a multi-faceted approach that addresses the underlying social and economic factors that can impact mental health, as well as the individual-level interventions that can help individuals cope with mental health issues. By working together to address these issues, we can create a more equitable and just society that promotes the mental health and wellbeing of all individuals.

The importance of ongoing efforts to break the stigma

Breaking the stigma around mental health is essential for promoting mental health and wellbeing for all individuals. Stigma can prevent individuals from seeking help for mental health issues, which can lead to more severe and long-term mental health problems.

Ongoing efforts to break the stigma surrounding mental health involve promoting education and awareness about mental health, as well as challenging negative attitudes and beliefs about mental illness. This includes encouraging individuals to seek help for mental health issues, and promoting the understanding that mental illness is a common and treatable health condition.

Breaking the stigma also involves addressing the social and cultural factors that contribute to negative attitudes towards mental illness, such as stereotypes and misinformation about mental health. This includes promoting media portrayals that accurately represent individuals with mental illness, and working towards reducing the discrimination and prejudice that can prevent individuals from seeking help for mental health issues.

By breaking the stigma surrounding mental health, we can promote a more supportive and accepting society that encourages individuals to seek help for mental health issues. This can lead to earlier intervention and treatment for mental health issues, which can improve outcomes and promote better mental health and wellbeing for all individuals. Overall, ongoing efforts to break the stigma surrounding mental health are essential for promoting a more equitable and just society that prioritizes mental health and wellbeing for all.

The need for ongoing research and innovation in mental health

Ongoing research and innovation in mental health are critical for advancing our understanding of mental health and improving outcomes for individuals with mental health issues. There is still much that we do not know about the causes and mechanisms of mental illness, and ongoing research is necessary to continue to uncover new insights and develop new treatments and interventions.

Research can also help to identify new risk factors for mental illness, as well as protective factors that can promote mental health and resilience. This information can be used to develop new prevention and early intervention strategies that can help to prevent the onset of mental health issues or reduce the severity of symptoms.

In addition, ongoing innovation is necessary to develop new and more effective treatments for mental health issues. This includes developing new medications, psychotherapies, and other interventions that are tailored to the unique needs of individuals with mental health issues.

Innovation is also needed to improve access to mental health services, particularly for marginalized populations who may face barriers to accessing care. This can involve developing new technologies or telehealth solutions that allow individuals to access mental health services from a distance, as well as developing new models of care that are more accessible and affordable.

The potential for a society that prioritizes mental health

A society that prioritizes mental health would be one in which individuals have access to high-quality mental health care and support services, and in which mental health and wellbeing are valued and promoted as important components of overall health and wellbeing.

This would involve addressing the underlying social and economic factors that can impact mental health, as well as promoting education and awareness about mental health and challenging negative attitudes and beliefs about mental illness.

In a society that prioritizes mental health, individuals would be encouraged to seek help for mental health issues without fear of stigma or discrimination. This would involve reducing the barriers that prevent individuals from accessing mental health care, such as stigma, lack of resources, and discrimination in healthcare settings. It would also involve promoting early intervention and treatment for mental health issues, as well as developing new prevention and early intervention strategies to reduce the risk of mental illness.

In addition, a society that prioritizes mental health would be one in which individuals have access to supportive environments and resources that promote mental health and wellbeing. This could involve promoting workplace policies that support mental health and wellbeing, such as flexible work arrangements and mental health days, as well as promoting community-level interventions that address the social determinants of mental health, such as access to education, employment, and healthcare.

Overall, a society that prioritizes mental health would be one in which individuals are able to lead healthy and fulfilling lives, free from the burden of mental illness. This would involve a commitment to ongoing education, awareness-raising, research, and innovation in mental health, as well as a commitment to promoting policies and interventions that address the underlying social and economic factors that can impact mental health. By prioritizing mental health, we can create a more equitable and just society that promotes the mental health and wellbeing of all individuals.

Conclusion:

In conclusion, mental health is an essential component of overall health and wellbeing, and it is essential that we prioritize it as such. By promoting mental health and wellbeing, we can help individuals to lead healthy and fulfilling lives, free from the burden of mental illness. This involves addressing the underlying social and economic factors that can impact mental health, promoting education and awareness about mental health, and challenging negative attitudes and beliefs about mental illness.

Mental health professionals play a critical role in promoting social justice and advancing mental health and wellbeing. By advocating for policies and interventions that promote mental health and wellbeing, mental health professionals can help to create a more equitable and just society that prioritizes the mental health and wellbeing of all individuals.

Ongoing efforts to break the stigma surrounding mental health and to invest in research and innovation in mental health are essential for advancing our understanding of mental health

and improving outcomes for individuals with mental health issues. By continuing to prioritize mental health and wellbeing, we can create a society that supports the mental health and wellbeing of all individuals, regardless of their background or circumstances. The importance of breaking the stigma surrounding mental illness
The potential benefits of prioritizing mental health for individuals and society
Call to action for ongoing efforts to reduce stigma and promote mental wellness